CANDIDA COOKBOOK

MAIN COURSE - Breakfast, Lunch, Dinner and Dessert Recipes to reset your health and treat candida

TABLE OF CONTENTS

BREAKFAST 7
BEKEDD EGGS WITH VEGETABLE HASH 7
RUTABAGA HASH 9
SAGE BREAKFAST PATTIES 11
COCONUT CEREAL 13
ZUCCHINI BREAD 15
BAKED EGGS WITH ONIONS 17
BIRCHER MUESLI 19
MORNING SOUFFLE 20
BUCKWHEAT MUFFFNIS 22
AVOCADO PANCAKES 24
GLUTEN- FREE WAFFLES 26
COCONUT GRANOLA 28
AVOCADO OMELET 30
YOGURT PARFAIT 31
BUCKWHEAT AND EGGS 32
SIMPLE OMELET 33
BUCHWHEAT PORRIDGE 34
COCONUT BREAD 35
GINGER CLOUDS 37
RHUBARB MUFFINS 38
LUNCH 41
BAKED LEMON SALMON 41
MEDITERRANENA BUDDA BOWL 43
RUTABAGA HASH 45

VEGAN CURRY 47

CAULIFLOWER WITH ROSEMARY 49

BRUSSELS SPROUTS 50

BREAD STUFFING 52

MOROCCAN STIR FRY 54

CAULIFLOWER FLORETS 56

ASIAN KEBABS 58

CITRUS FENNEL AND AVOCADO SALAD 60

KALE SALAD 61

GREEN SALAD 62

CANDIDA GREEN SALAD 63

KALE & MIXED GREENS SALAD 64

QUINOA SALAD 65

BRUSSELS SPROUT SALAD 66

CHINESE SALAD 67

BASIL & AVOCADO SALAD 68

MEDITERRANEAN SALAD 69

DINNER 71

VEGETABLE CABBAGE SOUP 71

CAULIFLOWER-GINGER SOUP 73

CELERY SOUP 75

ENERGY BOOSTING SOUP 77

CILANTRO SOUP 79

ONION SOUP 81

GINGER SOUP 82

CANDIDA DETOX SOUP 83

CANDIDA VEGETABLE SOUP	85
GARLIC-ASPARAGUS SOUP	87
SMOOTHIES	90
CANDIDA GREEN SMOOTHIE	90
CANDIDA FRIENDLY SMOOTHIE	92
ALKALINE SMOOTHIE	93
COCONUT SMOOTHIE	94
SHAMROCK SMOOTHIE	95
BLUEBERRY-PINEAPPLE SMOOTHIE	96
CANDIDA RASPBERRY SMOOTHIE	97
RASPBERRY-APPLE SMOOTHIE	98
CRANBERRY SMOOTHIE	99
ORANGE SMOOTHIE	100

Copyright 2019 by Noah Jerris - All rights reserved.

This document is geared towards providing exact and reliable information in regards to the topic and issue covered. The publication is sold with the idea that the publisher is not required to render accounting, officially permitted, or otherwise, qualified services. If advice is necessary, legal or professional, a practiced individual in the profession should be ordered.

- From a Declaration of Principles which was accepted and approved equally by a Committee of the American Bar Association and a Committee of Publishers and Associations.

In no way is it legal to reproduce, duplicate, or transmit any part of this document in either electronic means or in printed format. Recording of this publication is strictly prohibited and any storage of this document is not allowed unless with written permission from the publisher. All rights reserved.

The information provided herein is stated to be truthful and consistent, in that any liability, in terms of inattention or otherwise, by any usage or abuse of any policies, processes, or directions contained within is the solitary and utter responsibility of the recipient reader. Under no circumstances will any legal responsibility or blame be held against the publisher for any reparation, damages, or monetary loss due to the information herein, either directly or indirectly.

Respective authors own all copyrights not held by the publisher.

The information herein is offered for informational

purposes solely, and is universal as so. The presentation of the information is without contract or any type of guarantee assurance.

The trademarks that are used are without any consent, and the publication of the trademark is without permission or backing by the trademark owner. All trademarks and brands within this book are for clarifying purposes only and are the owned by the owners themselves, not affiliated with this document.

Introduction

Candida recipes for personal enjoyment but also for family enjoyment. You will love them for sure for how easy it is to prepare them.

BREAKFAST

BEKEDD EGGS WITH VEGETABLE HASH

Serves: **2**

Prep Time: *10* Minutes

Cook Time: *20* Minutes

Total Time: *35* Minutes

INGREDIENTS

- ¼ cup tomatoes
- ½ cup zucchini
- ½ cup yellow pepper
- 1 tablespoon olive oil
- 1 avocado
- 2 eggs
- salt

DIRECTIONS

1. Preheat the oven to 400 F
2. In a casserole dish add vegetables and drizzle olive oil over vegetables, mix well

3. Cut avocado in half, crack the eggs into each avocado half and sprinkle salt
4. Bake avocado and vegetables for 18-20 minutes or until vegetables are soft and eggs started to thicken
5. When ready remove from the oven and serve

RUTABAGA HASH

Serves: *4*
Prep Time: *10* Minutes
Cook Time: *20* Minutes
Total Time: *30* Minutes

INGREDIENTS

- 2 tablespoons olive oil
- 1 rutabaga
- ¼ cup red onion
- ¼ cup red pepper
- 1 tsp salt
- ¼ tsp pepper
- ¼ tsp dill

DIRECTIONS

1. In a skillet heat olive oil and sauté rutabaga for 4-5 minutes
2. Cover and cook until rutabagas are tender
3. Add red pepper, onion, paprika and sauté for 8-10 minutes

4. Add dill, pepper, salt and combine
5. When ready remove to a plate

SAGE BREAKFAST PATTIES

Serves: **6**

Prep Time: **10** Minutes

Cook Time: **15** Minutes

Total Time: **25** Minutes

INGREDIENTS

- 1 lb. turkey
- 1 tablespoon sage
- 1 tablespoon onions
- ¼ tsp thyme
- ¼ tsp garlic flakes
- ¼ tsp salt
- 1 tablespoon olive oil

DIRECTIONS

1. In a bowl add all ingredients and mix well
2. Divide mixture into 4-6 portions and form 4-6 solid patties
3. In a skillet heat olive oil and cook each one for 4-5 minutes per side

4. When ready remove from skillet and serve

COCONUT CEREAL

Serves: 2
Prep Time: 15 Minutes
Cook Time: 15 Minutes
Total Time: 30 Minutes

INGREDIENTS

- 1 cup almond flour
- ¼ tsp coconut
- 1 tsp cinnamon
- ¼ tsp salt
- ¼ tsp baking soda
- ¼ tsp vanilla extract
- 1 egg white
- 1 tablespoon olive oil

DIRECTIONS

1. Preheat the oven to 375 F
2. In a bowl combine baking soda, cinnamon, coconut, almond flour, salt and set aside

3. In another bowl combine vanilla extract, olive oil and mix well
4. In another bowl whisk the egg white and combine with vanilla extract mixture
5. Add almond flour to the vanilla extract mixture and mix well
6. Transfer dough onto a baking sheet and bake at 375 F for 10-15 minutes
7. When ready remove from the oven and serve

ZUCCHINI BREAD

Serves: *4*

Prep Time: *10* Minutes

Cook Time: *45* Minutes

Total Time: *55* Minutes

INGREDIENTS

- 1 zucchini
- 1 cup millet flour
- ½ cup almond flour
- ½ cup buckwheat flour
- 1 tsp baking powder
- ¼ tsp baking soda
- ¼ tsp salt
- ¼ cup almond milk
- 1 tsp apple cider vinegar
- 2 eggs
- ½ cup olive oil

DIRECTIONS

1. In a bowl combine almond flour, millet flour, buckwheat flour, baking soda, salt and mix well
2. In another bowl combine almond milk and apple cider vinegar
3. In a bowl beats eggs, add almond milk mixture and mix well
4. Add flour mixture to the almond mixture and mix well
5. Fold in zucchini and pour bread batter into pan
6. Bake at 375 F for 40-45 min
7. When ready remove from the oven and serve

BAKED EGGS WITH ONIONS

Serves: **2**

Prep Time: **10** Minutes

Cook Time: **20** Minutes

Total Time: **30** Minutes

INGREDIENTS

- 1 tablespoon olive oil
- 1 red bell pepper
- 1 red onion
- 1 cup tomatoes
- ¼ tsp salt
- ¼ tsp pepper
- 2 eggs
- parsley

DIRECTIONS

1. In a saucepan heat olive oil and sauté peppers and onions until soft
2. Add salt, pepper, tomatoes and cook for 4-5 minutes

3. Remove mixture and form 2 patties
4. Break the eggs into each pattie, top with parsley and place under the broiler for 5-6 minutes
5. When ready remove and serve

BIRCHER MUESLI

Serves: 2
Prep Time: 5 Minutes
Cook Time: 5 Minutes
Total Time: 10 Minutes

INGREDIENTS

- 1 cup coconut flakes
- ½ cup macadamia nuts
- 1 tablespoon chia seeds
- 1 tablespoon pumpkin seeds
- ¼ tsp cinnamon
- ¼ tsp ginger
- ¼ tsp nutmeg

DIRECTIONS

1. In a bowl combine all ingredients together
2. Place muesli in a container and refrigerate
3. When ready remove from the fridge and serve

MORNING SOUFFLE

Serves: **4**
Prep Time: **15** Minutes
Cook Time: **35** Minutes
Total Time: **50** Minutes

INGREDIENTS

- ¼ cup green chilies
- 1 cup avocado
- 1 cup grilled chicken
- 2 onions
- 4 eggs
- ½ cup milk
- 1 tablespoon coconut flour
- 1 tsp salt
- ¼ tsp pepper

DIRECTIONS

1. Scatter green chillies in the bottom of a baking dish

2. Add chicken, onions, avocado over green chillies and set aside
3. In another bowl combine coconut flour with eggs, pepper, salt and pour egg mixture over vegetables
4. Bake at 350 F for 30-35 minutes
5. When ready garnish with cilantro and serve

BUCKWHEAT MUFFFNIS

Serves: **8-12**

Prep Time: **10** Minutes

Cook Time: **15** Minutes

Total Time: **25** Minutes

INGREDIENTS

- 1 cup buckwheat groats
- ½ cup coconut flakes
- ¼ cup walnuts
- ¼ cup pumpkin seeds
- 1 tablespoon chia seeds
- ¼ cup flaxseed meal
- 1 tsp cinnamon
- 2 eggs
- 1 cup almond milk
- ¼ cup almond butter
- 2 packets powdered stevia
- 1 tablespoon vanilla extract

DIRECTIONS

1. In a bowl soak buckwheat groats overnight
2. In a bowl combine pumpkin seeds, buckwheat groats, chia seeds, cinnamon, salt, walnuts, flaxseed meal and coconut flakes
3. In a bowl combine almond milk, powdered stevia, eggs and combine
4. Combine almond mix mixture with buckwheat mixture and pour mixture into 8-12 muffins cups
5. Bake at 350 F for 12-15 minutes
6. When ready remove from the oven and serve

AVOCADO PANCAKES

Serves: **4**

Prep Time: **5** Minutes

Cook Time: **15** Minutes

Total Time: **20** Minutes

INGREDIENTS

- ¼ cup coconut flour
- ¼ tsp baking soda
- ¼ tsp salt
- 2 eggs
- ¼ cup almond milk
- ¼ avocado
- 2 green onions
- 1 tablespoon olive oil

DIRECTIONS

1. In a bowl combine dry ingredients with wet ingredients and mix well
2. In a skillet heat olive oil and pour ¼ batter and cook for 1-2 minutes per side

3. When ready remove to a place and serve with avocado slices

GLUTEN-FREE WAFFLES

Serves: **2**

Prep Time: **10** Minutes

Cook Time: **15** Minutes

Total Time: **25** Minutes

INGREDIENTS

- 3 egg whites
- 3 egg yolks
- ¼ cup coconut milk
- 1 tablespoon coconut oil
- 1 tsp vanilla extract
- ¼ tsp stevia
- ¼ cup almond flour
- ¼ tsp baking soda

DIRECTIONS

1. In a bowl combine wet ingredients with dry ingredients and mix well

2. Pour half of the batter into a waffle iron
3. And cook for 2-3 minutes or until the waffle is ready
4. Repeat the process for remaining batter
5. Serve waffle with applesauce

COCONUT GRANOLA

Serves: **6-8**

Prep Time: **10** Minutes

Cook Time: **20** Minutes

Total Time: **30** Minutes

INGREDIENTS

- 1 cup buckwheat groats
- 1 cup millet cereal
- 1 cup hazelnuts
- 1 cup coconut flakes
- ¼ cup flax seeds
- ¼ cup coconut oil
- 1 tsp vanilla extract
- 1 tsp powdered stevia
- 1 tsp cinnamon

DIRECTIONS

1. In a bowl combine all ingredients together, toss to combine

2. Spread granola mixture on a prepared baking sheet and bake at 350 F for 18-20 minutes
3. Remove from the oven and serve

AVOCADO OMELET

Serves: *1*
Prep Time: *10* Minutes
Cook Time: *15* Minutes
Total Time: *25* Minutes

INGREDIENTS

- 2 shallots
- 2 garlic cloves
- 2 eggs
- 1 avocado
- 5-6 black olives
- 1 tablespoon olive oil

DIRECTIONS

1. In a bowl crack eggs and beat them with parsley
2. In a skillet heat olive oil and sauté shallots and garlic until brown
3. Add the egg mixture and cook for 4-5 minutes
4. Add olives, avocado, fold and serve

YOGURT PARFAIT

Serves: *1*

Prep Time: *5* Minutes

Cook Time: *10* Minutes

Total Time: *15* Minutes

INGREDIENTS

- 1 apple
- Handful of walnuts
- 1 cup Greek yogurt
- pinch of cinnamon

DIRECTIONS

1. Chop the walnuts and cut the apples into thin slices
2. Layer them with the yogurt and sprinkle cinnamon
3. Serve when ready

BUCKWHEAT AND EGGS

Serves: 2
Prep Time: 5 Minutes
Cook Time: 15 Minutes
Total Time: 20 Minutes

INGREDIENTS

- ¼ cup buckwheat groats
- 2 eggs
- 1 tablespoon olive oil
- 1 spring onions
- handful of cilantros
- 1 tablespoon plain yogurt
- salt

DIRECTIONS

1. In a pan heat olive oil sauté onion for 2-3 minutes
2. Add cilantro, eggs and cook until eggs are cooked
3. Add salt, yogurt and serve

SIMPLE OMELET

Serves: *1*
Prep Time: *5* Minutes
Cook Time: *10* Minutes
Total Time: *15* Minutes

INGREDIENTS

- 2 eggs
- 2 tablespoons olive oil
- ¼ onion
- ¼ red pepper
- ¼ cup spinach
- salt

DIRECTIONS

1. In a skillet heat olive oil and sauté onions, spinach and peppers for 2-3 minutes
2. In a bowl beat eggs and add the eggs to the vegetables
3. Fold the omelet and place the omelet to a plate
4. Season and serve

BUCHWHEAT PORRIDGE

Serves: **4**

Prep Time: **10** Minutes

Cook Time: **30** Minutes

Total Time: **40** Minutes

INGREDIENTS

- ¼ cup buckwheat groats
- ¼ cup oats
- ½ cup almond milk
- 2 tablespoons coconut oil
- cinnamon

DIRECTIONS

1. Cook the buckwheat groats and set aside
2. Stir in coconut milk, cinnamon, coconut oil and mix well
3. Serve when ready

COCONUT BREAD

Serves: **4**

Prep Time: **10** Minutes

Cook Time: **30** Minutes

Total Time: **40** Minutes

INGREDIENTS

- ½ cup coconut flour
- ½ cup almond flour
- ½ cup coconut milk
- 4 eggs
- 2 tablespoons coconut oil
- ¼ tsp salt
- 1 tsp baking powder
- ¼ tsp vanilla extract

DIRECTIONS

1. In a blender add coconut oil, eggs, coconut flour coconut milk, almond flour, baking powder and blend until smooth

2. Pour mixture into a loaf pan and bake at 375 F for 25-30 minutes
3. When ready remove from the oven and serve

GINGER CLOUDS

Serves: *8-12*

Prep Time: *5* Minutes

Cook Time: *15* Minutes

Total Time: *20* Minutes

INGREDIENTS

- 2 egg whites
- 1 tsp powdered stevia
- 1 tablespoon vanilla extract
- 1 tsp ginger
- 1 ½ cup unsweetened coconut flakes

DIRECTIONS

1. Preheat the oven to 375 F
2. In a bowl whisk egg whites, add stevia, coconut flakes, ginger and vanilla extract
3. Mix well and drop tablespoon of size mounds of mixture onto a prepared baking sheet
4. Bake for 12-15 minutes at 325 F or until brown
5. When ready remove and serve

RHUBARB MUFFINS

Serves: **8-12**

Prep Time: **10** Minutes

Cook Time: **20** Minutes

Total Time: **30** Minutes

INGREDIENTS

- 1 cup buckwheat flour
- 1 cup almond flour
- 1 tsp cinnamon
- 1 tsp baking powder
- 1 tsp baking soda
- 2 eggs
- 1 tsp vanilla extract
- ½ cup almond milk
- ¼ tsp cinnamon
- 1 cup rhubarb

DIRECTIONS

1. **In a bowl add dry ingredients and mix well**

2. In another bowl add wet ingredients and mix well
3. Add wet ingredients to dry ingredients bowl and whisk to combine
4. Spoon batter into prepared muffin cups and bake for 18-20 minutes at 375 F
5. When ready remove from the oven and serve

LUNCH

BAKED LEMON SALMON

Serves: *1*

Prep Time: *10* Minutes

Cook Time: *20* Minutes

Total Time: *30* Minutes

INGREDIENTS

- 1 zucchini
- 1 onion
- 1 scallion
- 1 salmon fillet
- 1 tsp lemon zest
- 1 tsp olive oil
- Lemon slices

DIRECTIONS

1. Preheat the oven to 375 F
2. In a baking dish add zucchini, onion and sprinkle vegetables with salt and lemon zest

3. Lay salmon fillet and season with salt, lemon zest and olive oil
4. Bake at 375 F for 15-18 minutes
5. When ready remove from the oven and serve with lemon slices

MEDITERRANENA BUDDA BOWL

Serves: **1**

Prep Time: **10** Minutes

Cook Time: **10** Minutes

Total Time: **20** Minutes

INGREDIENTS

- 1 zucchini
- ¼ tsp oregano
- Salt
- 1 cup cooked quinoa
- 1 cup spinach
- 1 cup mixed greens
- ½ cup red pepper
- ¼ cup cucumber
- ¼ cup tomatoes
- parsley
- Tahini dressing

DIRECTIONS

1. In a skillet heat olive oil olive and sauté zucchini until soft and sprinkle oregano over zucchini
2. In a bowl add the rest of ingredients and toss to combine
3. Add fried zucchini and mix well
4. Pour over tahini dressing, mix well and serve

RUTABAGA HASH

Serves: 2
Prep Time: 10 Minutes
Cook Time: 20 Minutes
Total Time: 30 Minutes

INGREDIENTS

- 2 tablespoons olive oil
- 1 rutabaga
- ¼ cup onion
- ¼ cup red pepper
- 1 tsp salt
- ¼ tsp black pepper

DIRECTIONS

1. In a skillet heat olive oil and fry rutabaga for 3-4 minutes
2. Cook for another 5-6 minutes or until rutabaga is tender
3. Add onion, red pepper, black pepper, salt and stir to combine

4. Garnish with dill and serve

VEGAN CURRY

Serves: **4**
Prep Time: **10**   Minutes

Cook Time: **20**   Minutes

Total Time: **30**   Minutes

INGREDIENTS

- 1 tablespoon olive oil
- ¼ cup onion
- 2 stalks celery
- 1 garlic clove
- ¼ tsp coriander
- ¼ tsp cumin
- ¼ tsp turmeric
- ¼ tsp red pepper flakes
- 1 cauliflower
- 1 zucchini
- 2 tomatoes
- 1 tsp salt
- 1 cup vegetable broth
- 1 handful of baby spinach

- 1 tablespoon almonds
- 1 tablespoon cilantro

DIRECTIONS

1. In a skillet heat olive oil and sauté celery, garlic and onions for 4-5 minutes or until vegetables are tender
2. Add cumin, spices, coriander, cumin, turmeric red pepper flakes stir to combine and cook for another 1-2 minutes
3. Add zucchini, cauliflower, tomatoes, broth, spinach, water and simmer on low heat for 15-20 minutes
4. Add remaining ingredients and simmer for another 4-5 minutes
5. Garnish curry and serve

CAULIFLOWER WITH ROSEMARY

Serves: 2
Prep Time: 5 Minutes
Cook Time: 15 Minutes
Total Time: 20 Minutes

INGREDIENTS

- 1 cauliflower
- 1 tablespoon rosemary
- 1 cup vegetable stock
- 2 garlic cloves
- salt

DIRECTIONS

1. In a saucepan add cauliflower, stock and bring to a boil for 12-15 minutes
2. Blend cauliflower until smooth, add garlic, salt, rosemary and blend again
3. When ready pour in a bowl and serve

BRUSSELS SPROUTS

Serves: *2*
Prep Time: *10* Minutes
Cook Time: *20* Minutes
Total Time: *30* Minutes

INGREDIENTS

- 1 tablespoon olive oil
- 2 shallots
- 2 cloves garlic
- 1 lb. brussels sprouts
- 1 cup vegetable stock
- 4 springs thyme
- ¼ cup pine nuts

DIRECTIONS

1. In a pan heat olive oil and cook shallots until tender
2. Add garlic, sprouts, thyme, stock and cook for another 4-5 minutes

3. Cover and cook for another 10-12 minutes or until sprouts are soft
4. When ready add pine nuts and serve

BREAD STUFFING

Serves: **4**

Prep Time: **10** Minutes

Cook Time: **25** Minutes

Total Time: **35** Minutes

INGREDIENTS

- One loaf candida diet bread
- 1 tablespoon olive oil
- ¼ cup celery
- ¼ cup onion
- ¼ cup mushrooms
- ¼ cup leeks
- 1 tsp thyme
- ¼ tsp salt
- 1 cup vegetable broth

DIRECTIONS

1. Cut a loaf of candida diet bread cubes and place cubes aside

2. In a skillet heat olive oil add onion, celery, mushrooms and sauté for 5-10 minutes
3. Season with thyme, pepper, salt and stir to combine
4. Add vegetable mixture, broth, bread cubes and stir to combine
5. Place stuffing mixture into a casserole dish and bake for 12-15 minutes
6. Bake until golden brown and serve

MOROCCAN STIR FRY

Serves: 2
Prep Time: 10 Minutes
Cook Time: 20 Minutes
Total Time: 30 Minutes

INGREDIENTS

- ¼ cup onion
- 1 clove garlic
- 1 lb. ground turkey
- 1 tsp all spice
- 1 tsp cumin
- 1 tsp salt
- 2 cups cabbage
- 1 tablespoon mint
- 1 red bell pepper
- Zest of 1 lemon
- 1 tablespoon lemon juice
- plain yogurt
- pint leaves

DIRECTIONS

1. In a skillet heat olive oil and sauté garlic, onion until soft
2. Add cumin, pepper, salt, all spice, ground turkey and sauté for 8-10 minutes
3. Add cabbage, red bell pepper, pint leaves, lemon zest and sauté for 4-5 minutes
4. When ready garnish with mint leaves, yogurt and serve

CAULIFLOWER FLORETS

Serves: **2**

Prep Time: **10** Minutes

Cook Time: **30** Minutes

Total Time: **40** Minutes

INGREDIENTS

- 2 tablespoons olive oil
- 1 lb. cauliflower florets
- 1 tsp apple cider vinegar
- 1 tsp paprika
- ¼ tsp salt
- ¼ tsp onion powder
- ¼ tsp garlic powder
- 1 stalk celery
- 1 scallion
- 1 tablespoon parsley
- ranch dressing

DIRECTIONS

1. In a bowl add salt, onion powder, garlic powder, paprika, apple cider vinegar, olive oil and whisk to combine
2. Add cauliflower florets to the bowl and toss to coat
3. Place florets on a prepared baking sheet and bake at 375 F for 25-30 minutes
4. When ready remove from the oven and transfer to a place
5. Garnish with scallion, celery, parsley, drizzle ranch dressing and serve

ASIAN KEBABS

Serves: **8-12**

Prep Time: **10** Minutes

Cook Time: **20** Minutes

Total Time: **30** Minutes

INGREDIENTS

- 2 lb. steak
- 8-10 skewers
- Romain lettuce leaves
- Green onions

MARINADE

- ¼ cup coconut aminos
- 1 tablespoon water
- 1 tablespoon olive oil
- 2 cloves garlic
- 2 cloves onions
- 1 tablespoon sesame seeds
- 1 tsp pepper flakes

DIRECTIONS

1. Place all ingredients for the marinade in a bowl and mix well
2. Place steak cubes into the marinade bowl and let the meat marinade at least 8 hours
3. Preheat grill and place the steak kebabs on the grill
4. Cook for 4-5 minutes per side
5. When ready remove the kebabs from the gill and serve on lettuce leaves with green onions

CITRUS FENNEL AND AVOCADO SALAD

Serves: 2
Prep Time: 5 Minutes
Cook Time: 5 Minutes
Total Time: 10 Minutes

INGREDIENTS

- 5 cups baby greens
- 1 bulb fennel
- ¼ cup red onion
- 1 orange
- 1 grapefruit
- 6 cooked salmon fillet
- ¼ avocado
- ½ tsp garlic granules

DIRECTIONS

1. In a bowl mix all ingredients and mix well
2. Serve with dressing

KALE SALAD

Serves: 2
Prep Time: 5 Minutes
Cook Time: 5 Minutes
Total Time: 10 Minutes

INGREDIENTS

- 1 bunch kale
- Zest of 1 lemon
- ¼ cup tomatoes
- 1 tablespoon olive oil
- 1 tablespoon apple cider vinegar
- ½ cup pumpkin seeds
- ½ avocado

DIRECTIONS

1. In a bowl mix all ingredients and mix well
2. Serve with dressing

GREEN SALAD

Serves: 2
Prep Time: 5 Minutes
Cook Time: 5 Minutes
Total Time: 10 Minutes

INGREDIENTS

- 4 leaves kale
- 1 romaine heart
- 1 cup parsley leaves
- 1 cup cilantro leaves
- ¼ fennel bulb
- 1 carrot
- salad dressing

DIRECTIONS

1. In a bowl mix all ingredients and mix well
2. Serve with dressing

CANDIDA GREEN SALAD

Serves: 2
Prep Time: 5 Minutes
Cook Time: 5 Minutes
Total Time: 10 Minutes

INGREDIENTS

- ½ avocado
- 2 bolied eggs
- 2 tablespoons olive oil
- 2 tablespoons apple cider vinegar
- Oregano
- 1 cup spinach leaves
- 1 cucumber
- ½ cup asparagus
- ½ cup broccoli stems
- ½ avocado

DIRECTIONS

1. In a bowl mix all ingredients and mix well
2. Serve with dressing

KALE & MIXED GREENS SALAD

Serves: **2**

Prep Time: **5** Minutes

Cook Time: **5** Minutes

Total Time: **10** Minutes

INGREDIENTS

- 1 bunch kale
- 1 tablespoon olive oil
- 1 cup baby salad greens
- 1 carrot
- 1 small beet
- 1 celery stalk
- ¼ red bell pepper
- ¼ cup herbs
- ¼ steamed broccoli

DIRECTIONS

1. In a bowl mix all ingredients and mix well
2. Serve with dressing

QUINOA SALAD

Serves: 2
Prep Time: 5 Minutes
Cook Time: 5 Minutes
Total Time: 10 Minutes

INGREDIENTS

- 1 cooked chicken breast
- ¼ cup cooked quinoa
- 1 cup spinach
- 1 tomato
- ¼ cucumber
- 1 avocado
- 1 shallot
- 1 garlic clove
- 1 tablespoon olive oil

DIRECTIONS

1. In a bowl mix all ingredients and mix well
2. Serve with dressing

BRUSSELS SPROUT SALAD

Serves: 2

Prep Time: 5 Minutes

Cook Time: 5 Minutes

Total Time: 10 Minutes

INGREDIENTS

- 1 tablespoon olive oil
- 1 cup shallots
- ½ cup celery
- 1 clove garlic
- 6-8 brussels sprouts
- 1 tablespoon thyme leaves
- Herbs

DIRECTIONS

1. In a bowl mix all ingredients and mix well
2. Serve with dressing

CHINESE SALAD

Serves: 2
Prep Time: 5 Minutes
Cook Time: 5 Minutes
Total Time: 10 Minutes

INGREDIENTS

- 1 head cabbage
- 1 cup carrot
- ¼ cup scallions
- ¼ cup radishes
- ½ cup mint
- 1 cup cooked chicken breast

DIRECTIONS

1. In a bowl mix all ingredients and mix well
2. Serve with dressing

BASIL & AVOCADO SALAD

Serves: **2**

Prep Time: **5** Minutes

Cook Time: **5** Minutes

Total Time: **10** Minutes

INGREDIENTS

- 1 cup cooked chicken breast
- ¼ cup basil leaves
- 1 avocado
- 1 tablespoon olive oil
- ¼ tsp black pepper

DIRECTIONS

1. In a bowl mix all ingredients and mix well
2. Serve with dressing

MEDITERRANEAN SALAD

Serves: **2**
Prep Time: **5** Minutes
Cook Time: **5** Minutes
Total Time: **10** Minutes

INGREDIENTS

- 1 roasted chicken
- ¼ cup olive oil
- ¼ cup cilantro
- 1 red onion
- 1 head romaine lettuce
- ¼ lemon
- 1 cucumber
- 1 tomato

DIRECTIONS

1. In a bowl mix all ingredients and mix well
2. Serve with dressing

DINNER

VEGETABLE CABBAGE SOUP

Serves: **4-6**
Prep Time: **10** Minutes
Cook Time: **35** Minutes
Total Time: **45** Minutes

INGREDIENTS

- 1 leek
- 1 stalk celery
- 2 cups green beans
- 4 cups cabbage
- 1 cup cauliflower
- 1 cup broccoli
- 1 can tomato paste
- 1 tsp garlic
- 1 tsp basil
- ¼ tsp thyme leaves

DIRECTIONS

1. In a pot add green beans, celery, leek, cabbage and bring to a boil, simmer for low heat for 12-15 minutes
2. Add the remaining ingredients and simmer for another 12-15 minutes
3. When ready, pour soup into 2 prepared bowl, drizzle olive oil and serve with a pinch of pepper and herbs

CAULIFLOWER-GINGER SOUP

Serves: **4**

Prep Time: **10** Minutes

Cook Time: **25** Minutes

Total Time: **35** Minutes

INGREDIENTS

- 1 onion
- 1 stalk celery
- 1 cauliflower
- 1-inch piece ginger
- 2 cups vegetable stock
- ¼ tsp cumin
- ¼ tsp coriander
- ¼ tsp turmeric
- cilantro

DIRECTIONS

1. **In a bowl combine turmeric, cumin, coriander and set aside**

2. In a pot add ginger, celery, onion and simmer on low heat for 8-10 minutes
3. In a skillet add the spices, fry for 1-2 minutes and pour spices to the soup
4. Add cauliflower, vegetable stock, cover and simmer on low heat until cauliflower is fully cooked
5. When ready puree the soup until smooth
6. Pour soup into serving bowls and serve with cilantro

CELERY SOUP

Serves: **6**

Prep Time: **10** Minutes

Cook Time: **25** Minutes

Total Time: **35** Minutes

INGREDIENTS

- 1 onion
- 1 stalk celery
- 1 cauliflower
- 1 broccoli stalk
- 1 cup vegetable broth
- 1 cup water
- ¼ tsp garlic
- ¼ tsp turmeric

DIRECTIONS

1. In a pot add cauliflower, onion, celery, broth, garlic, turmeric and bring to a boil
2. Simmer on low heat for 12-15 minutes

3. Add broccoli, salt, and simmer for another 8-10 minutes or until broccoli is cooked
4. When ready remove from heat add salt and serve

ENERGY BOOSTING SOUP

Serves: **4**

Prep Time: **5** Minutes

Cook Time: **10** Minutes

Total Time: **15** Minutes

INGREDIENTS

- 1 onion
- 1 zucchini
- 1 cup broccoli florets
- 1 cup asparagus
- 1 cup collard leaves
- 1 tsp garlic
- 1 tsp olive oil
- 4 cups vegetable broth

DIRECTIONS

1. Place all ingredients in a pot and bring to a boil
2. When vegetables are soft puree soup until smooth

3. Add olive oil season and serve

CILANTRO SOUP

Serves: **4-6**
Prep Time: **10** Minutes
Cook Time: **20** Minutes
Total Time: **30** Minutes

INGREDIENTS

- 1 tablespoon butter
- 1 onion
- 1 stalk celery
- 1 clove garlic
- 4 zucchinis
- ¼ cup cilantro
- 2 cups vegetable broth
- ¼ cup scallions

DIRECTIONS

1. In a pot add garlic, celery, onion and sauté on low heat
2. Add remaining ingredients and bring to a boil

3. Simmer on low heat for 18-20 minutes
4. When vegetables are soft puree soup, season and serve

ONION SOUP

Serves: **2**

Prep Time: **5** Minutes

Cook Time: **5** Minutes

Total Time: **10** Minutes

INGREDIENTS

- 3 zucchinis
- 2 onions
- 2 garlic cloves
- 2 tablespoons olive oil

DIRECTIONS

1. Steam the onion and zucchini
2. Blend all ingredients until smooth
3. Pour soup into bowls and serve

GINGER SOUP

Serves: **2**

Prep Time: **5** Minutes

Cook Time: **10** Minutes

Total Time: **15** Minutes

INGREDIENTS

- 4 carrots
- 1 onion
- 1-inch piece ginger
- 1 can coconut milk
- 1 tsp cinnamon
- water

DIRECTIONS

1. In a saucepan add ginger, coconut milk, onion, carrots, water and bring to a boil
2. Simmer on low heat until vegetables are tender
3. Transfer soup to blender and blend until smooth
4. Pour soup into bowls, add a pinch of cinnamon and serve

CANDIDA DETOX SOUP

Serves: **4**
Prep Time: **10** Minutes
Cook Time: **35** Minutes
Total Time: **45** Minutes

INGREDIENTS

- 1 tablespoon olive oil
- 1 onion
- 1 stalk celery
- 1 yellow pepper
- 2 cloves garlic
- 2 cups green beans
- 2 cups vegetable stock
- 1 tsp basil
- ¼ tsp thyme
- 1 tsp salt
- 2 cups kale
- parsley

DIRECTIONS

1. In a pot heat olive oil and sauté celery, onion, garlic and bell pepper for 3-4 minutes
2. Ad green beans, vegetable stock, tomatoes, spices and remaining ingredients
3. Simmer on low heat for 22-25 minutes
4. When ready remove from heat, top with parsley and serve

CANDIDA VEGETABLE SOUP

Serves: **4-6**

Prep Time: **10** Minutes

Cook Time: **55** Minutes

Total Time: **65** Minutes

INGREDIENTS

- 2 onions
- 1 kale
- 4 stalks celery
- 4 garlic cloves
- 1 tsp salt
- Spices
- 8 cups water
- 1 tsp herbs de Provence
- ¼ tsp turmeric

DIRECTIONS

1. In a pot add all ingredients and bring to a boil
2. Cover and simmer on low heat for 45-50 minutes

3. When vegetables are tender remove soup from heat and blend soup until smooth
4. Pour soup into 2 prepare bowls, garnish with cilantro and serve

GARLIC-ASPARAGUS SOUP

Serves: **4**

Prep Time: **10** Minutes

Cook Time: **35** Minutes

Total Time: **45** Minutes

INGREDIENTS

- 1 tablespoon olive oil
- ¼ cup red onion
- 1 lb. asparagus
- ¼ lb. broccoli
- 4 garlic cloves
- 4 cups vegetable broth
- 1 tablespoon lemon juice
- 1 tablespoon tarragon

DIRECTIONS

1. In a pot heat olive oil and sauté onion, asparagus and broccoli for 5-6 minutes
2. Add broth and simmer for another 20-30 minutes or until vegetables are tender

3. Transfer soup to a blender and blend until smooth
4. Scoop the soup into bowls, drizzle with lemon juice, tarragon and olive oil
5. Serve when ready

SMOOTHIES

CANDIDA GREEN SMOOTHIE

Serves: **1**
Prep Time: **5** Minutes

Cook Time: **5** Minutes

Total Time: **10** Minutes

INGREDIENTS

- 12 oz. nondairy milk
- 1 cup spinach
- ¼ avocado
- 4 strawberries
- 1 tablespoon chia seeds
- ¼ tsp cinnamon
- 1 cup ice

DIRECTIONS

1. **In a blender place all ingredients and blend until smooth**

2. Pour smoothie in a glass and serve

CANDIDA FRIENDLY SMOOTHIE

Serves: *1*
Prep Time: *5* Minutes
Cook Time: *5* Minutes
Total Time: *10* Minutes

INGREDIENTS

- 1 cup water
- 2 cups spinach
- 1 cup romaine lettuce
- 1 cup cucumber
- 1 green apple
- 1 tablespoon lemon juice
- pinch of cinnamon

DIRECTIONS

1. In a blender place all ingredients and blend until smooth
2. Pour smoothie in a glass and serve

ALKALINE SMOOTHIE

Serves: *1*
Prep Time: *5* Minutes
Cook Time: *5* Minutes
Total Time: *10* Minutes

INGREDIENTS

- ½ cup coconut cream
- 1 cup baby spinach
- 1 avocado
- ¼ cucumber
- 1 tsp lime zest
- 1 cup ice

DIRECTIONS

1. In a blender place all ingredients and blend until smooth
2. Pour smoothie in a glass and serve

COCONUT SMOOTHIE

Serves: *1*

Prep Time: *5* Minutes

Cook Time: *5* Minutes

Total Time: *10* Minutes

INGREDIENTS

- 1 cup unsweetened coconut milk
- ¼ cup coconut milk
- 1 tablespoon peanut butter
- 1 tsp chia seeds
- 1 tsp vanilla extract

DIRECTIONS

1. In a blender place all ingredients and blend until smooth
2. Pour smoothie in a glass and serve

SHAMROCK SMOOTHIE

Serves: *1*
Prep Time: *5* Minutes
Cook Time: *5* Minutes
Total Time: *10* Minutes

INGREDIENTS

- 1 cucumber
- ½ avocado
- pinch of cinnamon
- 1 handful of peppermint leaves
- ½ cup kale leaves

DIRECTIONS

1. In a blender place all ingredients and blend until smooth
2. Pour smoothie in a glass and serve

BLUEBERRY-PINEAPPLE SMOOTHIE

Serves: 1
Prep Time: 5 Minutes
Cook Time: 5 Minutes
Total Time: 10 Minutes

INGREDIENTS

- 1 cup blueberries
- 1 cup pineapple
- 1 banana
- 4 oz. almond milk
- 1 cup ice

DIRECTIONS

1. In a blender place all ingredients and blend until smooth
2. Pour smoothie in a glass and serve

CANDIDA RASPBERRY SMOOTHIE

Serves: *1*
Prep Time: *5* Minutes
Cook Time: *5* Minutes
Total Time: *10* Minutes

INGREDIENTS

- 1 cup raspberries
- 1 mango
- 1 cup baby spinach
- 1 cup ice
- 1 cup watermelon

DIRECTIONS

1. In a blender place all ingredients and blend until smooth
2. Pour smoothie in a glass and serve

RASPBERRY-APPLE SMOOTHIE

Serves: *1*

Prep Time: 5 Minutes

Cook Time: 5 Minutes

Total Time: *10* Minutes

INGREDIENTS

- 1 cup raspberries
- 1 apple
- 1 pear
- 1 carrot
- 1 cup watermelon
- 1 cup ice

DIRECTIONS

1. In a blender place all ingredients and blend until smooth
2. Pour smoothie in a glass and serve

CRANBERRY SMOOTHIE

Serves: *1*
Prep Time: *5* Minutes
Cook Time: *5* Minutes
Total Time: *10* Minutes

INGREDIENTS

- ½ cup cranberry juice
- 1 apple
- 1 cup baby spinach
- 1 carrot
- 1 cup ice

DIRECTIONS

1. In a blender place all ingredients and blend until smooth
2. Pour smoothie in a glass and serve

ORANGE SMOOTHIE

Serves: **1**

Prep Time: **5** Minutes

Cook Time: **5** Minutes

Total Time: **10** Minutes

INGREDIENTS

- 1 orange
- 1 cup kale
- 1 banana
- 2 oz. almond milk
- 1 cup ice
- ½ apple

DIRECTIONS

1. In a blender place all ingredients and blend until smooth
2. Pour smoothie in a glass and serve

THANK YOU FOR READING THIS BOOK!

Printed in Great Britain
by Amazon